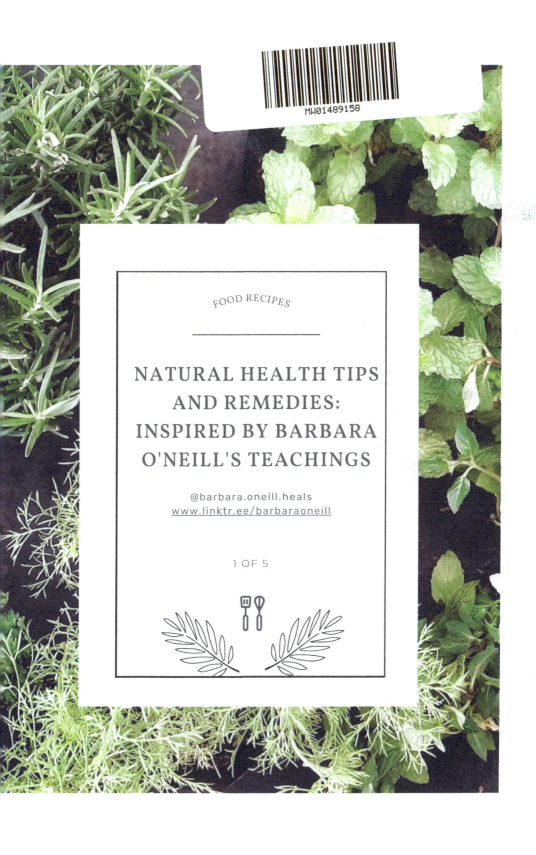

FOOD RECIPES

NATURAL HEALTH TIPS AND REMEDIES: INSPIRED BY BARBARA O'NEILL'S TEACHINGS

@barbara.oneill.heals
www.linktr.ee/barbaraoneill

1 OF 5

BARBARA ONEILL GENERAL TIPS

E-BOOK 1

TIPS AND REMEDIES EBOOK: INSPIRED BY
BARBARA O'NEILL'S TEACHINGS

@BARBARA.ONEILL.HEALS

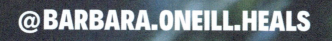

Hydration: Drink plenty of water throughout the day to stay hydrated and support bodily functions. Celtic salt in water helps the water go into the cell.

Barbara O'Neill Teachings

Mindful Eating: Paying attention to what you eat and how you eat can support digestion and promote a healthy relationship with food.

Positive Mindset: Cultivating a positive outlook and managing negative thoughts can contribute to overall mental and emotional well-being.

Plant-Based Nutrition: Following a diet rich in whole, plant-based foods is considered a foundational remedy for supporting overall well-being and preventing various health issues.

Hydration: Drinking plenty of water throughout the day is a fundamental remedy for maintaining overall health and supporting bodily functions.

Positive Social Connections: Maintaining healthy relationships and connections with loved ones contributes to emotional well-being.

Sleep Hygiene: Prioritizing quality sleep through consistent sleep schedules, a comfortable sleep environment, and relaxation techniques can enhance overall health.

Sunshine and Fresh Air: Spending time outdoors in natural sunlight and fresh air can have positive effects on mood, vitamin D levels, and overall vitality.

Exercise and Movement: Engaging in regular physical activity, such as walking, yoga, or stretching, is recommended for maintaining physical health and boosting mood.

Meditation and Relaxation: Practicing meditation, deep breathing, and other relaxation techniques can help manage stress, improve mental clarity, and promote a sense of calm.

Hydrotherapy: Hydrotherapy techniques, such as alternating hot and cold water applications, can stimulate circulation and support the body's natural healing processes.

Castor Oil Packs: Applying castor oil-soaked cloths to specific areas of the body is believed to help with detoxification, relaxation, and promoting healing.

Herbal Teas: Various herbal teas, such as chamomile, peppermint, and nettle, are often recommended for their potential health benefits, including relaxation and digestion support.

Ginger and Lemon Tea: A warm drink made from fresh ginger and lemon can help soothe digestion, support the immune system, and provide comfort during cold seasons.

Epsom Salt Baths: Epsom salt baths can be used to relax muscles, promote detoxification, and provide a calming effect on the body.

Herbal Remedies: Exploring the potential benefits of various herbs, such as echinacea, elderberry, and garlic, can support immune health and well-being.

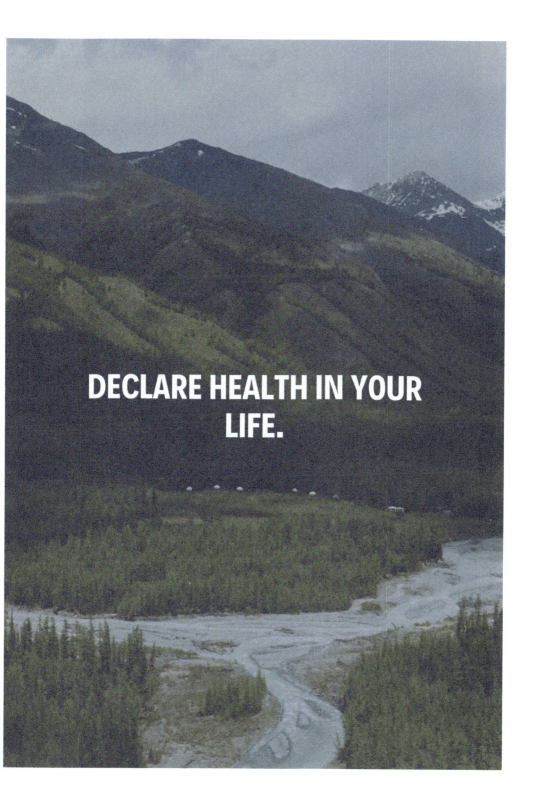

"Believe in your body's innate ability to heal. Your body is a remarkable instrument that can restore itself when given the right tools."– Barbara O'Neill

HEALTH AND WELLBEING

Barbara O'Neill's Teachings: A Holistic Approach to Health and Well-Being
In a world that often promotes quick fixes and isolated solutions, Barbara O'Neill's teachings stand as a refreshing beacon of holistic health wisdom. As a renowned health educator, O'Neill's approach embraces the interconnectedness of mind, body, and spirit, emphasizing natural remedies, nourishing nutrition, and mindful living. Her teachings, rooted in decades of experience, have resonated with countless individuals seeking comprehensive well-being.
The Holistic Philosophy: Mind, Body, and Spirit Unite
At the core of Barbara O'Neill's teachings is the understanding that true health is a result of nurturing the entire self—mind, body, and spirit. This holistic philosophy acknowledges that our mental and emotional states play a profound role in our physical well-being. O'Neill's approach encourages us to recognize the mind-body connection and to address both physical and emotional health to achieve true vitality.
Nourishing Nutrition: The Foundation of Wellness
Barbara O'Neill emphasizes the importance of nourishing our bodies with whole, unprocessed foods. She advocates for a plant-based diet rich in fruits, vegetables, whole grains, nuts, and seeds. O'Neill's teachings highlight the benefits of consuming nutrient-dense foods that provide essential vitamins, minerals, and antioxidants. Her advice aligns with research suggesting that such a diet can reduce the risk of chronic diseases and promote overall longevity.
Natural Remedies: Harnessing Nature's Healing Power
In line with her holistic approach, O'Neill champions the use of natural remedies for common ailments. Her teachings explore the healing properties of herbs, essential oils, and holistic practices. From soothing herbal teas to the potential benefits of aromatherapy, she empowers individuals to tap into nature's pharmacy for healing and wellness support.
Stress Management: Cultivating Resilience Through Mindfulness
Modern life's demands often lead to stress and burnout. Barbara O'Neill's teachings offer practical strategies for managing stress and cultivating emotional resilience. She guides individuals toward mindfulness practices, deep breathing exercises, and techniques that promote relaxation. By addressing stress from a holistic perspective, she helps individuals find balance and restore a sense of calm.
Detoxification: Supporting the Body's Natural Cleansing
Barbara O'Neill's teachings on detoxification emphasize supporting the body's natural processes rather than endorsing extreme cleansing methods. She advocates for clean eating, staying hydrated, and incorporating foods that aid the liver and kidneys in eliminating toxins. O'Neill's approach underscores the importance of gradual, sustainable changes that promote long-term well-being.
Exercise and Movement: Energizing the Body
Physical activity is another cornerstone of Barbara O'Neill's teachings. She encourages regular exercise that aligns with individual preferences and capabilities. From brisk walking to rebounding and yoga, her teachings highlight the importance of keeping the body active for circulation, energy, and overall vitality.
Holistic Living: A Lifelong Journey
Barbara O'Neill's teachings remind us that achieving and maintaining well-being is an ongoing journey. Her approach is not about quick fixes but about cultivating a balanced, mindful lifestyle that supports optimal health for the long term. By embracing her teachings, individuals can foster a deeper connection with their bodies, their environment, and the power of natural remedies.
In a world where health advice can be fragmented and overwhelming, Barbara O'Neill's teachings provide a holistic roadmap for achieving vitality and well-being. Her wisdom offers a return to the fundamentals—nourishing nutrition, natural remedies, stress management, and a mindful approach to living—that can transform lives and empower individuals to take charge of their health in a meaningful and sustainable way.

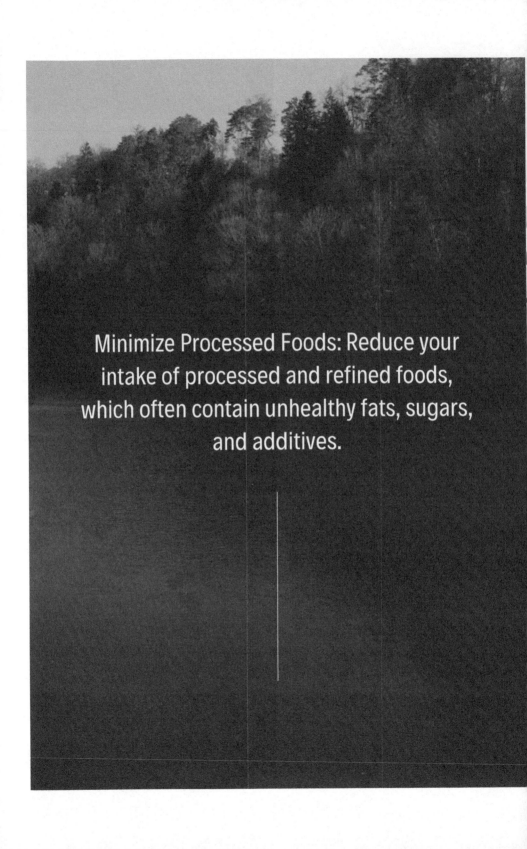

Minimize Processed Foods: Reduce your
intake of processed and refined foods,
which often contain unhealthy fats, sugars,
and additives.

99

"Listen to your body. It often gives subtle signals about what it needs for optimal health."- Barbara O'Neill

@barbara.oneill.heals

LIKE, FOLLOW FOR MORE

DIET TIPS

1. Plant–Based Foods: Barbara O'Neill emphasizes a diet rich in plant–based foods. This includes vegetables, fruits, whole grains, legumes, nuts, and seeds.
2. Raw and Cooked Vegetables: Incorporating a variety of colorful vegetables, both raw and cooked, provides essential vitamins, minerals, and antioxidants.
3. Whole Grains: Whole grains like brown rice, quinoa, psyllium, and whole wheat provide fiber, energy, and essential nutrients.
4. Fruits: A variety of fresh fruits can provide natural sweetness, vitamins, and minerals. Berries, citrus fruits, apples, and bananas are common choices.
5. Legumes: Beans, lentils, chickpeas, and other legumes are excellent sources of plant–based protein, fiber, and nutrients.
6. Nuts and Seeds: These provide healthy fats, protein, and various nutrients. Examples include almonds, walnuts, chia seeds, and flaxseeds.
7. Plant–Based Proteins: Plant–based protein sources like tofu, tempeh, and seitan can be included for additional protein in the diet.
8. Healthy Fats: Unsaturated fats from sources like avocados, olive oil, and nuts are often encouraged in moderation.
9. Herbal Teas: Herbal teas like chamomile, peppermint, and ginger can be enjoyed for their potential health benefits.
10. Hydration: Staying hydrated by drinking water throughout the day is essential for overall well–being.
11. Whole and Unprocessed Foods: Barbara O'Neill's philosophy often emphasizes avoiding or minimizing processed foods, refined sugars, and artificial additives.
12. Portion Control: Practicing portion control and mindful eating is important to avoid overeating.

Many remedies and supplements can also be found on our instagram link in bio
@barbara.oneill.heals

More recipe books and remedies will be available for all exclusive subscribers to our instagram page

Want quality supplements or herbs? You may also visit the shop > linktr.ee/barbaraoneill

{Embrace a Plant–Based Diet: Prioritize whole plant foods like vegetables, fruits, legumes, nuts, and seeds. These foods are rich in nutrients and contribute to overall health.}

WHAT TO AVOID

Barbara O'Neill advocates for a holistic and natural approach to health and wellness, which includes avoiding certain foods that are considered less beneficial for overall well-being. While I can't provide verbatim quotes from her, I can give you an overview of the types of foods she often suggests avoiding or minimizing in one's diet:

Processed Foods:
    Processed foods often contain additives, preservatives, artificial flavors, and excessive amounts of salt and sugar. Barbara recommends reducing or eliminating these from the diet.

Refined Sugar:
    Highly refined sugars found in sugary snacks, sodas, and desserts can lead to spikes and crashes in blood sugar levels. She often suggests reducing intake of these items.

Trans Fats and Hydrogenated Oils:
    These unhealthy fats are commonly found in fried foods, commercially baked goods, and certain packaged snacks. Barbara advises avoiding these fats in favor of healthier fats like those found in nuts, seeds, and avocados.

Artificial Sweeteners:
    Barbara often suggests avoiding artificial sweeteners due to concerns about their potential impact on health. Instead, she recommends using natural sweeteners like honey or maple syrup in moderation.

Refined Grains:
    Refined grains, such as white flour, lack the fiber and nutrients found in whole grains. She recommends choosing whole grains like brown rice, quinoa, and whole wheat.

Highly Processed Meats:
    Highly processed meats like sausages, hot dogs, and certain deli meats can contain preservatives and additives. She advises opting for lean, minimally processed meats or exploring plant-based protein sources.

Excessive Dairy:
    While dairy can be part of a balanced diet for some individuals, Barbara suggests moderating its consumption, especially if there are concerns about lactose intolerance or dairy allergies.

Artificial Additives and Preservatives:
    Barbara emphasizes the importance of choosing whole, natural foods without artificial colors, flavors, and preservatives. These additives can potentially have negative effects on health.

Sodas and Sweetened Beverages:
    Sugary sodas and drinks often provide empty calories and contribute to blood sugar imbalances. She suggests opting for water, herbal teas, or freshly made fruit juices.

GMO Foods:
    Barbara may recommend avoiding or reducing the consumption of genetically modified organisms (GMO) foods due to concerns about their potential impact on health and the environment.

Many remedies and supplements can also be found on our instagram link in bio
@barbara.oneill.heals

More recipe books and remedies will be available for all exclusive subscribers to our instagram page

Want quality supplements or herbs? You may also visit the shop > linktr.ee/barbaraoneill

"

"Nature holds the key to our well-
being. Embrace the healing power
of herbs, plants, and natural
remedies." - Barbara O'Neill

WEIGHT

Barbara O'Neill's approach to weight loss and obesity centers around holistic lifestyle changes, mindful eating, and fostering a healthy relationship with food. Her recommendations emphasize sustainable practices that support overall well-being. It's important to consult with a healthcare professional before making significant changes to your diet or exercise routine, especially if you have underlying health conditions. Here are some of Barbara O'Neill's suggested remedies and advice for weight loss or obesity:

1. Nourishing Nutrition:
Focus on whole, nutrient-dense foods such as fruits, vegetables, whole grains, lean proteins, and healthy fats.
Avoid or minimize processed foods, sugary snacks, and refined carbohydrates.
Practice mindful eating by paying attention to hunger cues and eating slowly to recognize when you're full.

2. Portion Control:
Be mindful of portion sizes to prevent overeating. Use smaller plates and bowls to help manage portion sizes visually.

3. Balanced Meals:
Aim for balanced meals that include a combination of carbohydrates, proteins, and fats. This helps stabilize blood sugar levels and keeps you satiated.

4. Hydration:
Stay hydrated by drinking water throughout the day. Sometimes, our bodies confuse thirst with hunger. Use celtic salt in water to ensure absorption

5. Regular Physical Activity:
Engage in regular exercise that you enjoy, whether it's walking, swimming, dancing, or yoga. Consistency is key for long-term success.

6. Mindful Movement:
Incorporate movement into your daily routine, such as taking the stairs, walking to nearby destinations, or practicing light stretching.

7. Emotional Eating Awareness:
Recognize emotional triggers that lead to overeating. Practice finding healthier ways to cope with stress, boredom, or other emotions.

8. Quality Sleep:
Prioritize adequate sleep as it supports hormone regulation and helps prevent overeating due to fatigue.

9. Stress Management:
Practice stress-reduction techniques like deep breathing, meditation, and spending time in nature. Stress can impact eating behaviors.

10. Supportive Environment: - Surround yourself with positive influences that encourage healthy choices. Share your goals with friends or family who can provide support.

11. Self-Compassion: - Approach weight loss with self-compassion and kindness. Avoid harsh self-criticism and focus on progress rather than perfection.

suggested products in our bio link : MCT Oil, Ashwaganda, Chromium, Celtic Salt
Barbara O'Neill's teachings emphasize that weight loss should be approached as a journey toward overall well-being. Rather than relying on fad diets or extreme measures, her holistic approach encourages a balanced and sustainable lifestyle that supports gradual, long-term weight management. Remember that individual responses may vary, and consulting a healthcare professional or registered dietitian can provide personalized guidance based on your unique needs and circumstances.

99

"Food is the foundation of health. Choose nourishing, whole foods that provide your body with the nutrients it needs to thrive."- Barbara O'Neill

99

"Practice mindfulness and gratitude. Being present and thankful enhances your overall sense of well-being."- Barbara O'Neill

STRESS / DEPRESSION

Barbara O'Neill's holistic approach to addressing stress and depression focuses on a combination of lifestyle adjustments, natural remedies, and mindful practices. It's important to note that her recommendations should be considered as part of a comprehensive approach and should not replace professional medical advice. Here are some remedies that she might suggest:

1. Mindfulness and Meditation:
   - Engage in mindfulness meditation to cultivate present-moment awareness and reduce stress. Meditation practices can help calm the mind and promote emotional well-being.

2. Deep Breathing Exercises:
   - Practice deep breathing techniques to activate the body's relaxation response. Slow, deep breaths can help alleviate stress and anxiety.

3. Herbal Teas:
   - Certain herbal teas like chamomile, lemon balm, and passionflower are known for their calming properties. Sipping on these teas can have a soothing effect on the nervous system.

4. Aromatherapy:
   - Use essential oils like lavender, bergamot, and frankincense through aromatherapy. These oils can be diffused, inhaled, or used in diluted form for massage to promote relaxation.

5. Physical Activity:
   - Engage in regular physical activity to release endorphins, which are natural mood enhancers. Activities like walking, yoga, and tai chi can be particularly beneficial.

6. Balanced Nutrition:
   - Consume a balanced diet rich in nutrient-dense foods. rich in omega-3s, whole grains, leafy greens, and nuts can support brain health and mood regulation.

7. Herbal Supplements:
   - Certain herbal supplements, such as St. John's wort and rhodiola rosea, have been traditionally used to support emotional well-being. However, it's important to consult a healthcare professional before using any supplements, as they can interact with medications.

8. Sunlight Exposure:
   - Spend time outdoors in natural sunlight, as it can boost mood and regulate circadian rhythms. Sunlight exposure helps stimulate the production of serotonin, a neurotransmitter associated with happiness.

9. Positive Social Interactions:
   - Foster positive connections with friends, family, and support groups. Social interactions can provide emotional support and a sense of belonging.

10. Sleep Hygiene: - Prioritize quality sleep by establishing a consistent sleep schedule, creating a comfortable sleep environment, and practicing relaxation techniques before bed.

11. Limiting Stimulants and Processed Foods: - Reduce or eliminate caffeine, sugary foods, and processed snacks, as they can contribute to mood swings and energy crashes.

Barbara O'Neill's approach emphasizes that addressing stress and depression requires a multifaceted approach that encompasses the mind, body, and spirit. It's important to seek guidance from a qualified healthcare professional if you're experiencing persistent or severe symptoms of stress or depression. These remedies can complement traditional therapies but should not be considered a substitute for professional medical care.

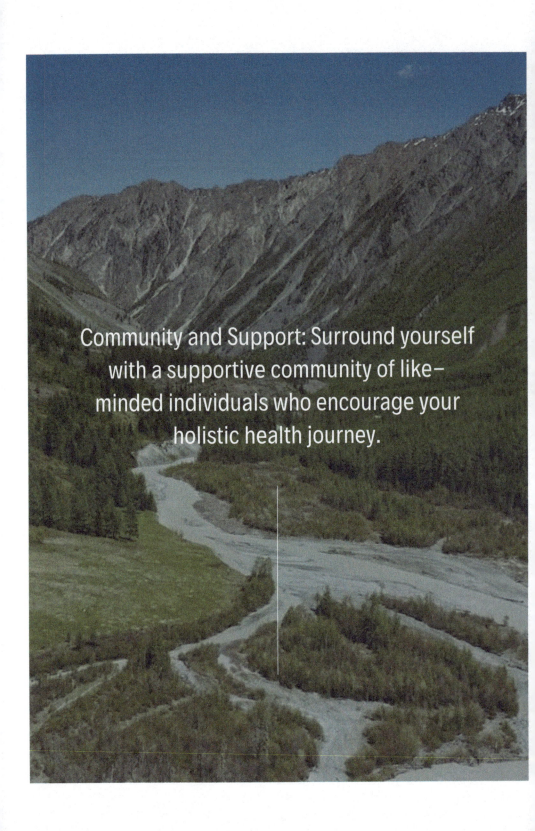

Community and Support: Surround yourself with a supportive community of like-minded individuals who encourage your holistic health journey.

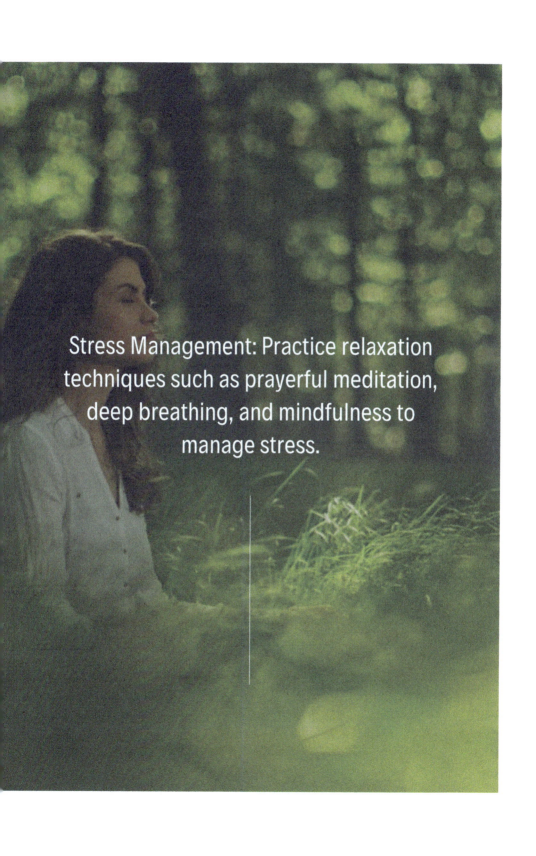

Stress Management: Practice relaxation techniques such as prayerful meditation, deep breathing, and mindfulness to manage stress.

"But I will restore you to health and heal your wounds,' declares the LORD." – Jeremiah 30:17

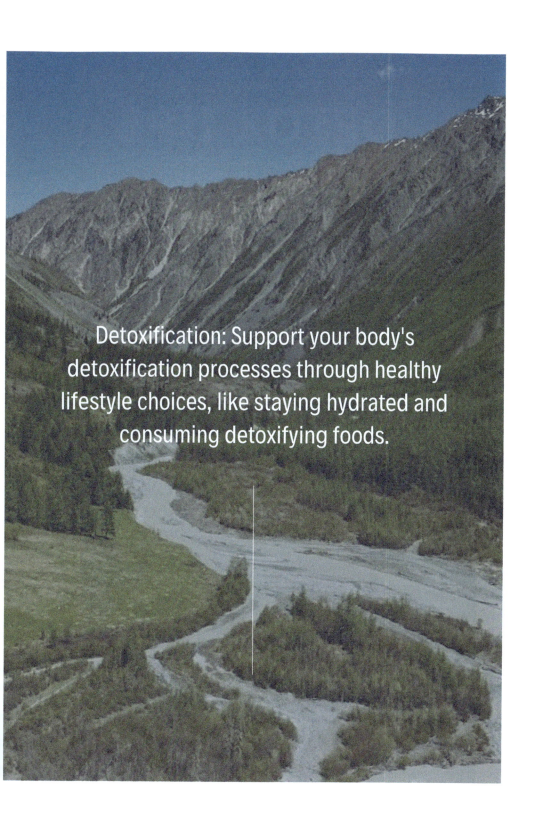

Detoxification: Support your body's detoxification processes through healthy lifestyle choices, like staying hydrated and consuming detoxifying foods.

DETOX TIPS

Barbara O'Neill often emphasizes the importance of supporting the body's natural detoxification processes through healthy lifestyle choices. Her approach to detoxing is holistic, focusing on dietary and lifestyle changes to assist the body in eliminating toxins and promoting overall well-being. While I can't provide verbatim quotes from her, I can offer a general overview of her ideas on detoxification and how to approach it:

Clean Eating:
  Barbara O'Neill recommends adopting a clean, plant-based diet rich in whole foods. This includes fruits, vegetables, whole grains, nuts, seeds, and legumes. These foods provide essential nutrients and fiber that aid in digestion and elimination.

Hydration:
  Staying well-hydrated is crucial for detoxification. Drinking clean, filtered water supports the body's natural cleansing processes by aiding in the removal of waste and toxins.

Avoid Processed Foods:
  Processed foods, which often contain additives, preservatives, and artificial ingredients, can burden the body's detoxification pathways. Barbara advises minimizing or eliminating these from the diet.

Fiber-Rich Foods:
  Foods high in dietary fiber, such as whole grains, vegetables, and legumes, promote regular bowel movements and help eliminate waste and toxins from the body.

Supportive Herbs:
  Barbara often recommends incorporating herbs with detoxifying properties into your diet. Examples include dandelion, milk thistle, burdock root, and nettle. These herbs are believed to support liver and kidney function.

Exercise:
  Engaging in regular physical activity, such as brisk walking, rebounding, or yoga, helps stimulate circulation, lymphatic flow, and sweating, which can aid in the elimination of toxins.

Stress Management:
  Chronic stress can impact the body's detoxification processes. Barbara suggests practicing relaxation techniques like deep breathing, meditation, and mindfulness to manage stress.

Sauna and Skin Care:
  Sweating through activities like sauna sessions can help release toxins through the skin. Using natural skin care products and dry brushing may also support healthy skin and detoxification.

Adequate Sleep:
  Quality sleep is crucial for the body's repair and detoxification processes. Barbara emphasizes getting enough restorative sleep each night.

Mind-Body Connection:
  Addressing emotional well-being is also a part of detoxification. Nurturing a positive mindset, managing emotional stress, and fostering a sense of joy and balance can contribute to overall health.

Many remedies and supplements can also be found on our instagram link in bio @barbara.oneill.heals

More recipe books and remedies will be available for all exclusive subscribers to our instagram page

Want quality supplements or herbs? You may also visit the shop > linktr.ee/barbaraoneill

CASTOR OIL PACK

Ingredients:
- High-quality cold-pressed castor oil
- Unbleached and organic flannel cloth or wool fabric
- Plastic wrap or a large plastic bag
- Hot water bottle or heating pad
- Old towel or cloth

Instructions:

1. Prepare the Materials:
   - Cut the flannel cloth into a size large enough to cover the targeted area of your body.
   - Fold the cloth into multiple layers to make a pack that's not too thin or too thick.
   - Place an old towel or cloth underneath you to protect surfaces from oil stains.

2. Apply Castor Oil:
   - Pour a sufficient amount of castor oil onto the cloth, enough to saturate it but not to the point of dripping.
   - Lie down on your back in a comfortable spot, such as a bed or couch.

3. Apply the Pack:
   - Place the castor oil-soaked cloth onto the targeted area of your body. Common areas include the abdomen, liver, or other areas in need of support.
   - Cover the cloth with plastic wrap or place it in a large plastic bag to prevent oil from getting on your bedding or clothing.

4. Apply Heat:
   - Place a hot water bottle or heating pad on top of the plastic-covered pack. The heat helps the castor oil penetrate the skin and promotes relaxation.
   - Make sure the heat is comfortable; it shouldn't be too hot to cause discomfort.

5. Relax and Rest:
   - Lie down and relax for about 30 to 60 minutes. You can use this time to meditate, read, or simply unwind.
   - It's a good idea to have a calming activity to make the most of this time.

6. Removing the Pack:
   - After the desired time, remove the pack and gently wipe off any excess oil using a clean cloth.
   - You can store the castor oil-soaked cloth in a glass container for future use. Keep it in the refrigerator.

7. Cleanse the Skin:
   - Wash the area where you applied the pack with mild soap and water to remove any remaining oil.

Frequency:
- Castor oil packs can be used 2-3 times per week or as recommended by a health professional.

Many remedies and supplements can also be found on our instagram link in bio @barbara.oneill.heals

More recipe books and remedies will be available for all exclusive subscribers to our instagram page

Want quality supplements or herbs? You may also visit the shop > linktr.ee/barbaraoneill

BARBARA ONEILL
GENERAL TIPS

@BARBARA.ONEILL.HEALS

{"True healing encompasses the body, mind, and spirit. When these elements are in harmony, optimal health is achieved."–Barbara O'Neill}

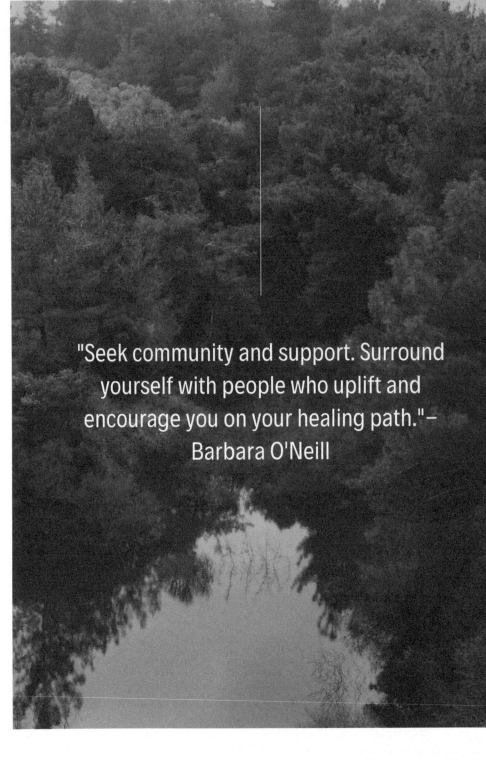

"Seek community and support. Surround yourself with people who uplift and encourage you on your healing path."– Barbara O'Neill

99

"Connect with nature regularly.
Spending time outdoors
rejuvenates the spirit and
supports overall health." – Barbara
O'Neill

@barbara.oneill.heals

LIKE, FOLLOW FOR MORE

BARBARA ONEILL
GENERAL TIPS

"

"Treat your body as a temple. Fuel it with nourishing foods, keep it active, and nurture it with love."- Barbara O'Neill

TEA RECIPES

. Immune-Boosting Herbal Tea: Ingredients:

- 1 teaspoon echinacea root
- 1 teaspoon elderberry
- 1 teaspoon dried rosehips
- 1 teaspoon dried thyme
- 2 cups water
- Honey (optional)

Instructions:
1. In a small pot, bring the water to a gentle simmer.
2. Add the echinacea root, elderberry, rosehips, and thyme.
3. Allow the herbs to simmer for about 10 minutes.
4. Strain the tea into cups.
5. Sweeten with honey if desired.
6. Enjoy this immune-boosting blend that's rich in antioxidants.

2. Calming Lemon Balm Lavender Tea: Ingredients:

- 1 tablespoon dried lemon balm leaves
- 1 teaspoon dried lavender flowers
- 2 cups hot water
- Lemon or honey (optional)

Instructions:
1. Place the dried lemon balm leaves and lavender flowers in a teapot or cup.
2. Pour hot water over the herbs and let steep for about 5-7 minutes.
3. Strain the tea into cups.
4. Add a squeeze of lemon or a drizzle of honey if desired.
5. Experience the calming effects of this aromatic blend.

3. Digestive Ginger Peppermint Tea: Ingredients:

- 1-inch piece of fresh ginger, sliced
- 1 teaspoon dried peppermint leaves
- 2 cups boiling water
- Honey (optional)

Instructions:
1. Place the sliced ginger and peppermint leaves in a teapot or cup.
2. Pour boiling water over the herbs and steep for about 5-7 minutes.
3. Strain the tea into cups.
4. Sweeten with honey if desired.
5. Enjoy the soothing and digestive benefits of this blend.

4. Cleansing Dandelion Nettle Tea: Ingredients:

- 1 teaspoon dried dandelion root
- 1 teaspoon dried nettle leaves
- 2 cups hot water
- Lemon (optional)

Instructions:
1. Combine the dried dandelion root and nettle leaves in a teapot or cup.
2. Pour hot water over the herbs and steep for about 10-15 minutes.
3. Strain the tea into cups.
4. Add a squeeze of lemon if desired.
5. Experience the potential cleansing properties of this herbal blend.

Herbal Remedies: Explore the benefits of herbal remedies for various ailments. Herbal teas and natural supplements can support your well-being.

FLU BOMB

Immune–Boosting Flu Bomb Tonic:

Ingredients:

1 inch piece of fresh ginger, grated
2 cloves of garlic, minced
1 lemon, juiced
1 tablespoon raw honey
1 pinch cayenne pepper (optional)
1 cup warm water
Instructions:

In a mug, combine the grated ginger, minced garlic, lemon juice, and raw honey.
If using cayenne pepper, add a pinch to the mug.
Pour warm water over the ingredients in the mug.
Stir well to combine all the ingredients.
Let the tonic steep for a few minutes to infuse the flavors.
Sip the tonic slowly while it's still warm.
This tonic combines ingredients that are often associated with immune–boosting properties.
Ginger and garlic are known for their potential anti–inflammatory and immune–supportive
effects. Lemon provides vitamin C, while raw honey can have antibacterial and soothing
properties. The cayenne pepper, if used, might provide an additional kick and potential
circulation support.

Many remedies and supplements can also be found on our instagram link in bio
@barbara.oneill.heals

More recipe books and remedies will be available for all exclusive subscribers to our instagram
page

Want quality supplements or herbs? You may also visit the shop > linktr.ee/barbaraoneill

GINGER TEA

3. Ginger Turmeric Wellness Tea: Ingredients:
- 1-inch piece of fresh ginger, sliced
- 1/2 teaspoon ground turmeric
- Dash of black pepper (to enhance turmeric absorption)
- Hot water
- Honey (optional)

Instructions:
1. Place the sliced ginger in a teapot or cup.
2. Add the ground turmeric and a dash of black pepper.
3. Pour hot water over the herbs and spices and let steep for about 5–7 minutes.
4. Strain the tea into cups.
5. Sweeten with honey if desired.
6. Sip and enjoy the potential immune–boosting benefits of this warming tea.

Mass produced milk is processed. If the dairy we consume was fed to a calf it would die. - Barbara O'Neill

Many remedies and supplements can also
be found on our instagram link in bio
@barbara.oneill.heals

More recipe books and remedies will be
available for all exclusive subscribers to our
instagram page

Want quality supplements or herbs? You
may also visit the shop >
linktr.ee/barbaraoneill

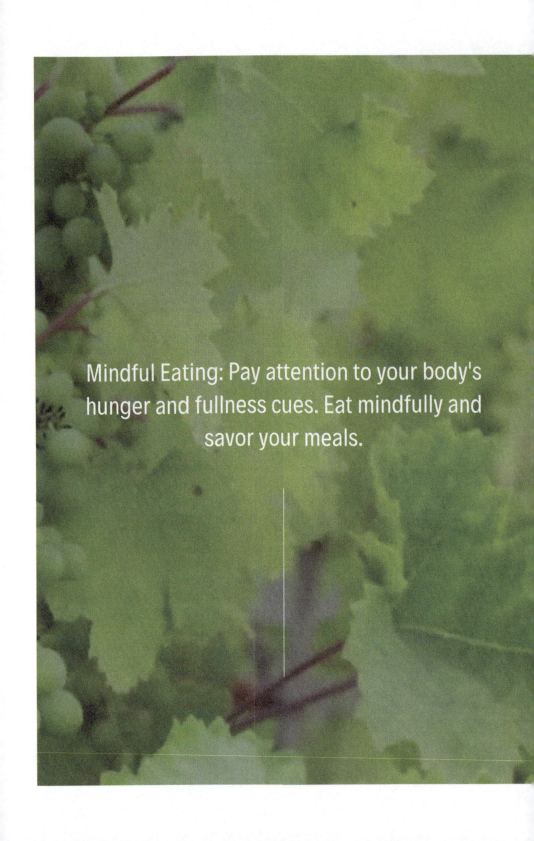

Mindful Eating: Pay attention to your body's hunger and fullness cues. Eat mindfully and savor your meals.

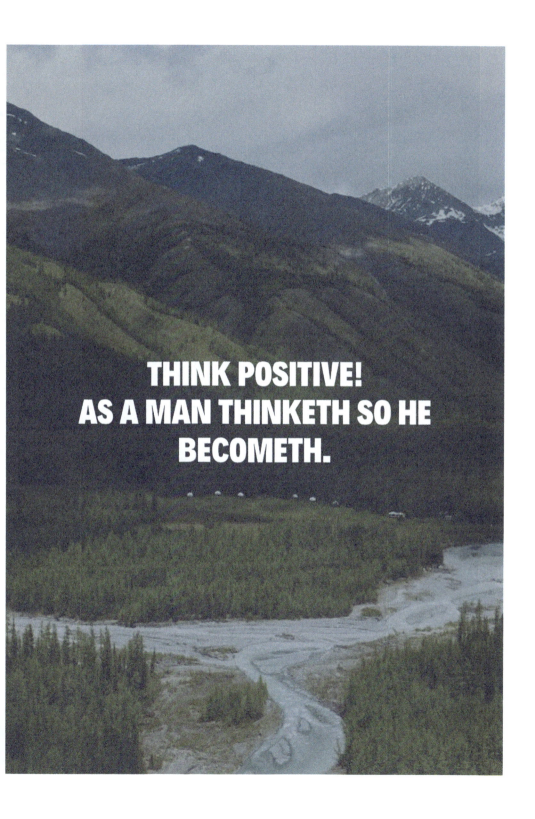

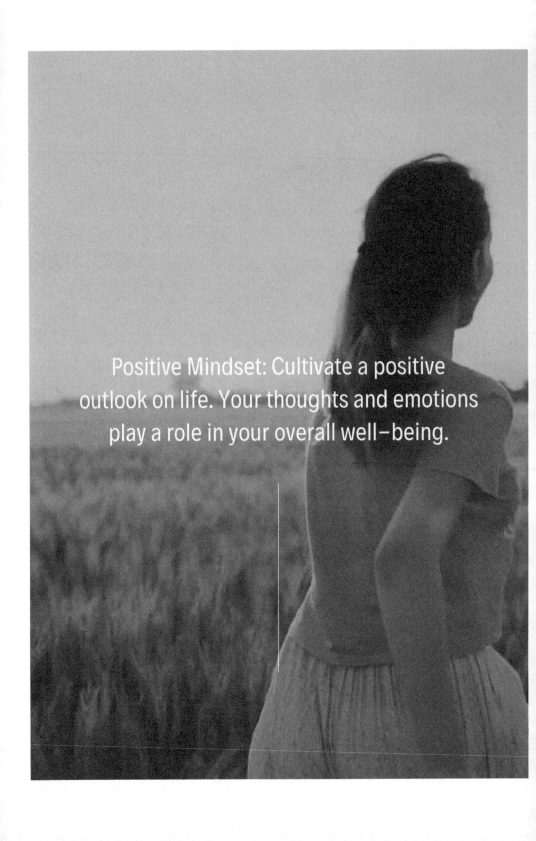

Positive Mindset: Cultivate a positive outlook on life. Your thoughts and emotions play a role in your overall well-being.

REMEDIES

Barbara O'Neill often emphasizes a holistic approach to addressing illnesses and health concerns. While I can provide general advice based on holistic principles, it's important to note that individual cases can vary, and you should consult with a healthcare professional for personalized guidance. Here are some common illnesses and general remedy advice that align with Barbara O'Neill's holistic approach:

Common Cold and Immune Support:

Barbara might recommend staying hydrated, consuming vitamin C–rich foods (such as citrus fruits), and using immune–supporting herbs like echinacea or elderberry. Rest and proper sleep are crucial for recovery.

Digestive Issues:

For digestive discomfort, she might suggest avoiding processed foods, consuming ginger or peppermint tea for soothing effects, and eating probiotic–rich foods like yogurt to support gut health. Consider probiotic supplements. Check for mineral balances.

Stress and Anxiety:

Barbara often emphasizes relaxation techniques such as deep breathing, meditation, or mindfulness to manage stress. Engaging in regular physical activity, spending time in nature, and fostering a positive mindset are also encouraged.

Insomnia:

To promote better sleep, she might recommend establishing a bedtime routine, avoiding screen time before bed, avoid caffeine, and practicing relaxation techniques. Herbal teas like chamomile or valerian root could be considered, but it's essential to consult a healthcare professional. Breathing techniques or try melatonin or check hormones.

Allergies:

Barbara might suggest reducing exposure to allergens, staying hydrated, consuming anti–inflammatory foods (such as omega–3 fatty acids from fish), and using herbal remedies like nettles or butterbur (under professional guidance). Avoiding top allergens like wheat, dairy, nuts, eggs, may benefit. Using curcumin supplements may bring down inflamation.

Skin Issues (Eczema, Acne, etc.):

She might recommend avoiding processed foods, dairy, and foods high in refined sugars. Increasing intake of nutrient–rich foods like fruits, vegetables, and healthy fats can support skin health. Herbal remedies like calendula cream might be suggested, bicarb or boron bath, also castor oil and MCT on our instagram page may help.

Headaches:

Barbara might advise identifying triggers like certain foods, dehydration, or stress. Staying hydrated, managing stress, and ensuring proper sleep are important. Peppermint oil or lavender oil aromatherapy could also be considered.

Joint Pain and Inflammation:

She might suggest consuming anti–inflammatory foods like turmeric, ginger, and omega–3 fatty acids. Incorporating gentle exercise, such as swimming or yoga, and staying hydrated are also important. Try boron or magnesium or charcoal on our link in bio.

Low Energy and Fatigue:

Barbara often recommends a nutrient–dense diet, including complex carbohydrates, protein, and healthy fats. Avoiding processed foods and incorporating regular exercise can also boost energy levels. Consider our vitamin b liquid or iron supplement on our link in our bio.

Urinary Tract Infections (UTIs):

Drinking plenty of water and unsweetened cranberry juice might be advised to support urinary tract health. Herbal remedies like uva ursi might be considered, but consultation with a healthcare professional is crucial. Try boron on our instagram link.

Remember that these recommendations are general and based on holistic principles. Individual cases can vary, and it's important to seek advice from healthcare professionals, naturopathic practitioners, or registered dietitians when addressing specific health concerns. Additionally, if you have any underlying health conditions or are on medication, it's crucial to consult a healthcare professional before trying any remedies or making significant lifestyle changes.

Many remedies and supplements can also be found on our instagram link in bio @barbara.oneill.heals

More recipe books and remedies will be available for all exclusive subscribers to our instagram page. Want quality supplements or herbs? You may also visit the shop > linktr.ee/barbaraoneill

99

"Remember that health is a journey, not a destination. Every positive choice you make contributes to your well-being."- Barbara O'Neill

99

"Physical activity is medicine for the body and mind. Find movement that brings you joy and make it a regular part of your life."- Barbara O'Neill

@barbara.oneill.heals

LIKE, FOLLOW FOR MORE

EXCERCISE TIPS

HITT Training!

Rebounder (Mini Trampoline):

- How to Use:
    a. Purchase a high-quality mini trampoline (rebounder). see our link   found on our instagram link in bio @barbara.oneill.heals You may also visit the shop > linktr.ee/barbaraoneill

    a. Start with gentle bouncing, gradually increasing the intensity as your fitness improves.
    b. Bounce for 5-20 minutes per session, depending on your fitness level.
    c. Incorporate gentle movements like jogging in place, bouncing on one foot, or light jumping jacks.
    d. Remember to warm up before and cool down after your rebounding session.
- Benefits: Rebounding is a low-impact exercise that can help improve lymphatic circulation, boost cardiovascular health, strengthen muscles, and increase overall energy levels. It's also believed to support detoxification and stimulate various bodily systems.

Many remedies and supplements can also be found on our instagram link in bio @barbara.oneill.heals

More recipe books and remedies will be available for all exclusive subscribers to our instagram page

Want quality supplements or herbs? You may also visit the shop > linktr.ee/barbaraoneill

High-Intensity Interval Training (HIIT) Exercise Overview

High-Intensity Interval Training (HIIT) is a popular and effective workout technique that alternates between short bursts of intense exercise and periods of lower-intensity recovery or rest. This style of training is known for its efficiency in burning calories, improving cardiovascular fitness, and building muscular strength. HIIT workouts can be adapted to various fitness levels and goals, making them a versatile choice for those seeking time-efficient and challenging exercise routines. Here's an overview of HIIT training and how it works:

Key Components of HIIT:

1. Intervals: HIIT workouts are structured around intervals of high-intensity exercise followed by periods of low-intensity exercise or rest. The high-intensity intervals challenge your cardiovascular system and muscles, while the recovery intervals allow you to catch your breath and prepare for the next intense round.
2. Intensity: During the high-intensity intervals, you exert maximum effort to elevate your heart rate and push your limits. This can involve exercises like sprinting, jumping, or high-impact movements.
3. Recovery: The recovery intervals are active rest periods where you continue to move at a lower intensity. This could involve jogging, walking, or slower bodyweight exercises.

Benefits of HIIT:

- Efficient Calorie Burn: HIIT workouts burn a significant amount of calories in a short time, making them effective for weight management and fat loss.
- Improved Cardiovascular Fitness: The alternating high-intensity and recovery periods challenge your cardiovascular system, enhancing your aerobic and anaerobic capacity.
- Time-Saving: HIIT workouts are typically shorter than traditional steady-state cardio sessions, making them ideal for individuals with busy schedules.
- Muscular Endurance and Strength: HIIT exercises often involve bodyweight movements or resistance exercises, which can improve muscular endurance and strength.
- Metabolic Boost: HIIT can elevate your metabolism post-workout, leading to continued calorie burn even after you've finished exercising.

Sample HIIT Workout:

Warm-Up: 5-10 minutes of light cardio and dynamic stretches.

Circuit:

1. Jump Squats: 20 seconds of intense jumping squats.
   o Recovery: 10 seconds of easy jogging in place.
2. Push-Ups: 20 seconds of rapid push-ups (modify if needed).
   o Recovery: 10 seconds of slow, controlled squats.
3. Burpees: 20 seconds of explosive burpees.
   o Recovery: 10 seconds of marching in place.
4. Mountain Climbers: 20 seconds of quick mountain climbers.
   o Recovery: 10 seconds of slow bodyweight lunges.

Repeat the circuit 3-4 times.

Cool-Down: 5-10 minutes of static stretches and deep breathing.

Remember, HIIT workouts can be tailored to your fitness level. Beginners might start with longer recovery intervals or lower-intensity exercises, gradually increasing intensity as fitness improves. Consult a healthcare professional before starting any new exercise program, especially if you have underlying health conditions or concerns.

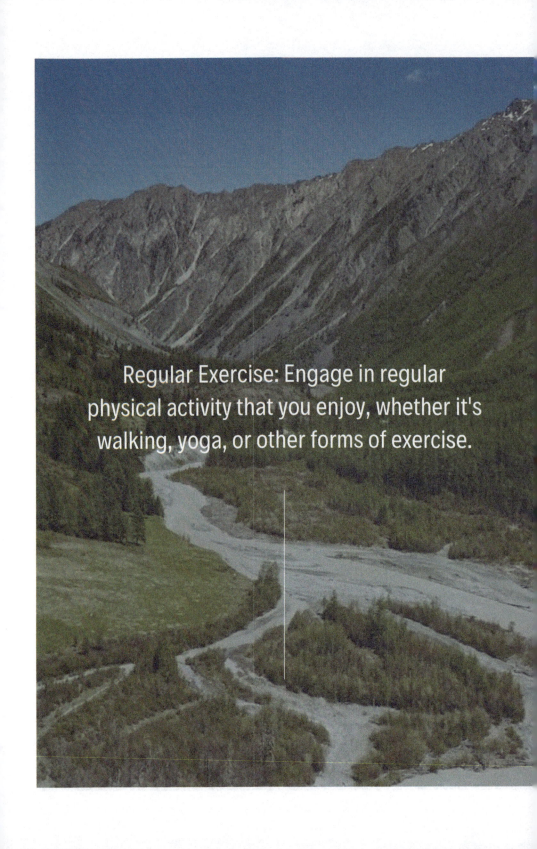

Regular Exercise: Engage in regular physical activity that you enjoy, whether it's walking, yoga, or other forms of exercise.

99

"Detoxify your body regularly. A clean body is a pathway to vitality and longevity." - Barbara O'Neill

LIKE, FOLLOW FOR MORE

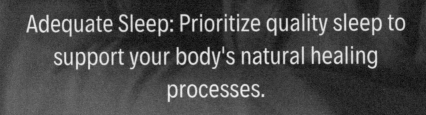

Adequate Sleep: Prioritize quality sleep to support your body's natural healing processes.

"Practice mindfulness and gratitude. Being present and thankful enhances your overall sense of well-being."- Barbara O'Neillearth-conservation causes.

99

"Choose happiness and positivity.
Cultivating a joyful outlook
contributes to a healthier life."-
Barbara O'Neill

@barbara.oneill.heals

LIKE, FOLLOW FOR MORE

SLEEP TIPS

Barbara O'Neill often provides holistic advice for improving sleep quality. While I can't provide verbatim quotes from her, I can offer you a collection of tips that align with her holistic approach to better sleep:

1. Establish a Sleep Routine:
   - Go to bed and wake up at the same time every day, even on weekends, to regulate your body's internal clock.
2. Create a Calming Bedtime Routine:
   - Engage in relaxing activities before bed, such as reading, gentle stretching, meditation, or deep breathing.
3. Limit Screen Time:
   - Reduce exposure to screens (phones, tablets, computers, TVs) at least an hour before bedtime. The blue light emitted by screens can interfere with the production of the sleep hormone melatonin.
4. Avoid Heavy Meals and Stimulants:
   - Refrain from consuming heavy, spicy, or large meals close to bedtime. Minimize caffeine and nicotine intake, especially in the afternoon and evening.
5. Create a Comfortable Sleep Environment:
   - Make your bedroom conducive to sleep by keeping it dark, quiet, and at a comfortable temperature. Consider using blackout curtains, earplugs, or a white noise machine if needed.
6. Limit Fluid Intake Before Bed:
   - Minimize drinking liquids close to bedtime to reduce the likelihood of waking up for bathroom trips during the night.
7. Regular Physical Activity:
   - Engage in regular exercise during the day, but avoid vigorous exercise close to bedtime, as it can be stimulating.
8. Relaxation Techniques:
   - Practice relaxation techniques such as meditation, deep breathing, or progressive muscle relaxation before bed to calm the mind and body.
9. Limit Napping:
   - If you have trouble sleeping at night, try to limit daytime napping, especially in the late afternoon.
10. Manage Stress:
    - Address stressors through healthy coping mechanisms, such as journaling, talking to a friend, or engaging in a hobby you enjoy.
11. Avoid Clock-Watching:
    - Constantly checking the time can increase anxiety about not being able to fall asleep. Consider removing visible clocks from your bedroom.
12. Consider Herbal Teas:
    - Some herbal teas like chamomile, valerian root, or passionflower may have calming effects that promote sleep. Consult a healthcare professional before using any herbal remedies.
13. Avoid Alcohol Before Bed:
    - While alcohol may initially make you feel drowsy, it can disrupt sleep cycles and lead to poorer sleep quality.
14. Natural Supplements:
    - Consult a healthcare professional before considering natural supplements like melatonin, magnesium, or certain herbs that are sometimes recommended to aid sleep.

Many remedies and supplements can also be found on our instagram link in bio @barbara.oneill.heals

More recipe books and remedies will be available for all exclusive subscribers to our instagram page

Want quality supplements or herbs? You may also visit the shop > linktr.ee/barbaraoneill

"Embrace the healing power of rest. Quality sleep is a cornerstone of good health."– Barbara O'Neill

HEART HEALTH

1. Heart-Healthy Diet:
   - Embrace a plant-based diet rich in fruits, vegetables, whole grains, legumes, and nuts. These foods provide essential nutrients that support heart health.
2. Omega-3 Fatty Acids:
   - Incorporate sources of omega-3 fatty acids, flaxseeds, chia seeds, and walnuts. These fats are beneficial for heart health.
3. Fiber-Rich Foods:
   - Consume foods high in soluble fiber, such as psyllium, beans, lentils, and fruits like apples and berries. Soluble fiber helps lower cholesterol levels.
4. Healthy Fats:
   - Opt for healthy fats from sources like olive oil, avocados, and nuts while minimizing saturated and trans fats.
5. Stress Management:
   - Practice stress-reduction techniques such as deep breathing, meditation, and yoga to promote relaxation and reduce the impact of stress on the heart.
6. Physical Activity:
   - Engage in regular aerobic exercise like brisk walking, swimming, or cycling to support cardiovascular health and improve circulation.
7. Maintain a Healthy Weight:
   - Aim for a healthy weight that aligns with your body's needs. Weight management contributes to overall heart health.
8. Blood Pressure Control:
   - Consume foods rich in potassium (e.g., bananas, leafy greens) and reduce sodium intake to help regulate blood pressure.
9. Antioxidant-Rich Foods:
   - Eat foods rich in antioxidants, such as colorful fruits and vegetables, to protect the heart from oxidative stress.
10. Hydration: - Stay well-hydrated with water, herbal teas, and naturally flavored water to support overall health.
11. Limit Refined Sugars and Processed Foods: - Reduce consumption of sugary snacks, sugary beverages, and processed foods, as they can contribute to inflammation and heart disease risk.
12. Mindful Eating: - Practice mindful eating by savoring meals, eating slowly, and paying attention to hunger and fullness cues.
13. Supportive Social Connections: - Cultivate positive relationships and connections with loved ones, which can have a positive impact on heart health.
14. Regular Health Checkups: - Schedule regular checkups with a healthcare professional to monitor blood pressure, cholesterol levels, and overall heart health.

Barbara O'Neill's holistic approach to heart health underscores the importance of making lifestyle choices that promote wellness from the inside out. While these suggestions are inspired by her teachings, it's crucial to work closely with healthcare professionals to address heart conditions, especially if you have existing heart issues or risk factors. These recommendations are not a substitute for medical advice but can complement a comprehensive heart health plan.

Cayenne pepper, great for heart health
and circulation- Barbara O'Neill

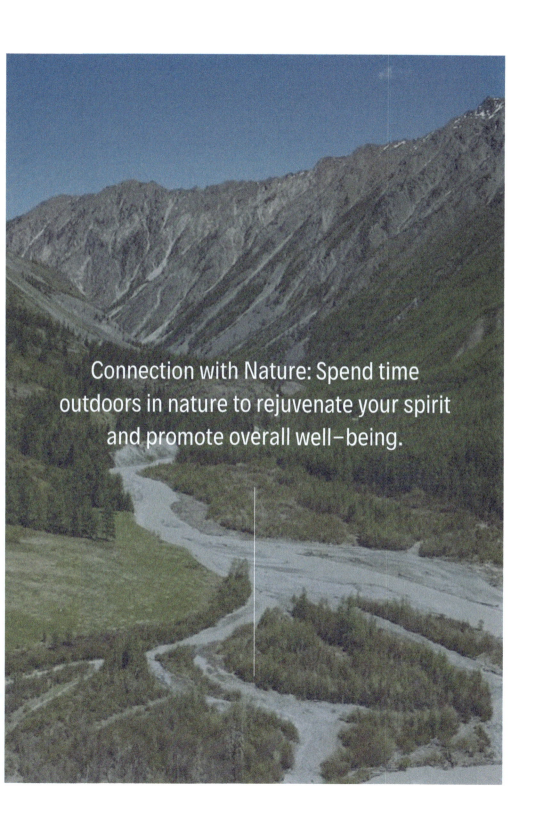

Connection with Nature: Spend time outdoors in nature to rejuvenate your spirit and promote overall well-being.

"Simplicity is key. Strive for balance in all aspects of your life, and avoid overcomplicating your health journey."– Barbara O'Neill

Many remedies and supplements can also be found on our instagram link in bio @barbara.oneill.heals

More recipe books and remedies will be available for all exclusive subscribers to our instagram page

Want quality supplements or herbs? You may also visit the shop > linktr.ee/barbaraoneill

SUPPLEMENTS

Barbara O'Neill often emphasizes obtaining nutrients from whole foods as a primary source of nutrition. However, in certain cases, she might recommend supplements to address specific health concerns or deficiencies. Here are some supplements that she might suggest, but remember to consult with a healthcare professional before adding any new supplements to your routine . More recipe books and remedies will be available for all exclusive subscribers to our instagram page. Want quality supplements or herbs? You may also visit the shop > linktr.ee/barbaraoneill

Vitamin D:

> Vitamin D is essential for bone health, immune function, and overall well-being. Some people may have limited sun exposure, leading to low vitamin D levels. A supplement might be recommended if deficiency is confirmed through blood tests.

Omega-3 Fatty Acids:

> Omega-3 fatty acids are known for their anti-inflammatory properties and potential benefits for heart and brain health. Plant-based supplements like flaxseed oil can provide these essential fatty acids.

Magnesium:

> Magnesium is involved in numerous bodily processes, including muscle function, nerve function, and energy production. Some individuals may benefit from magnesium supplements, especially if they have low dietary intake.

B Vitamins:

> B vitamins play a crucial role in energy metabolism, nerve function, and overall health. A B-complex supplement might be recommended for those with specific deficiencies or dietary restrictions.

Probiotics:

> Probiotics are beneficial bacteria that support gut health and immune function. They can be particularly useful for individuals with digestive issues or after a course of antibiotics.

Iron:

> Iron is essential for carrying oxygen in the blood. Individuals with iron-deficiency anemia might require iron supplements, but it's important to get tested before starting supplementation.

Vitamin C:

> Vitamin C is known for its antioxidant properties and its role in immune function. It might be recommended for individuals with a greater need for immune support.

Zinc:

> Zinc is involved in immune function, wound healing, and maintaining healthy skin. A zinc supplement might be suggested for those with low dietary intake or specific health needs.

Turmeric or Curcumin:

> Turmeric contains curcumin, a compound with anti-inflammatory and antioxidant properties. A supplement might be considered for its potential health benefits, but consuming turmeric in your diet is also valuable.

Multivitamins:

> In some cases, a high-quality multivitamin might be suggested to ensure a balanced intake of essential nutrients, especially for individuals with restricted diets.

Remember that supplements should not replace a balanced diet and healthy lifestyle. They are meant to complement your nutritional intake when specific deficiencies or health conditions exist. Before taking any supplements, it's important to consult with a healthcare professional, registered dietitian, or naturopathic practitioner to ensure they are appropriate for your individual needs and circumstances.

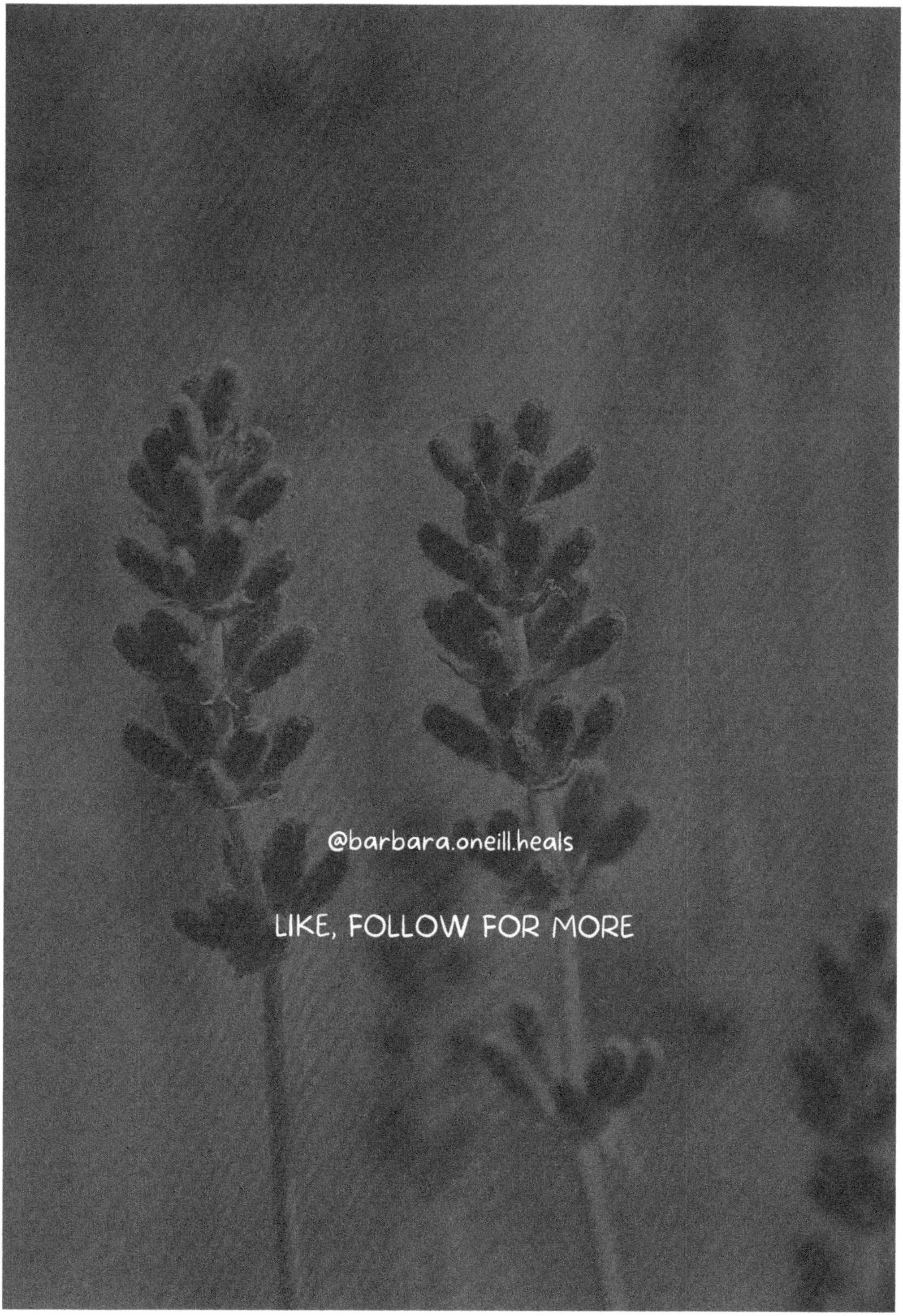
@barbara.oneill.heals
LIKE, FOLLOW FOR MORE

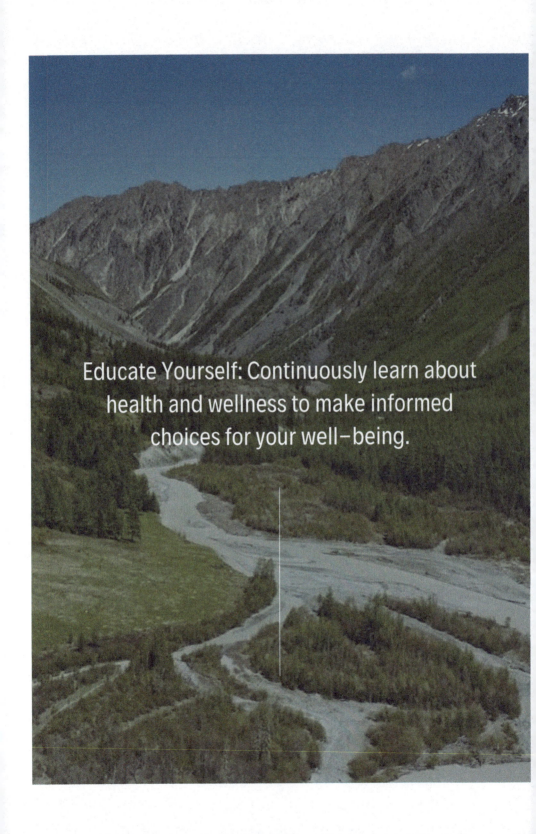

Educate Yourself: Continuously learn about health and wellness to make informed choices for your well-being.

99

"Remember that prevention is the best medicine. Take proactive steps to maintain good health and prevent illness."– Barbara O'Neill

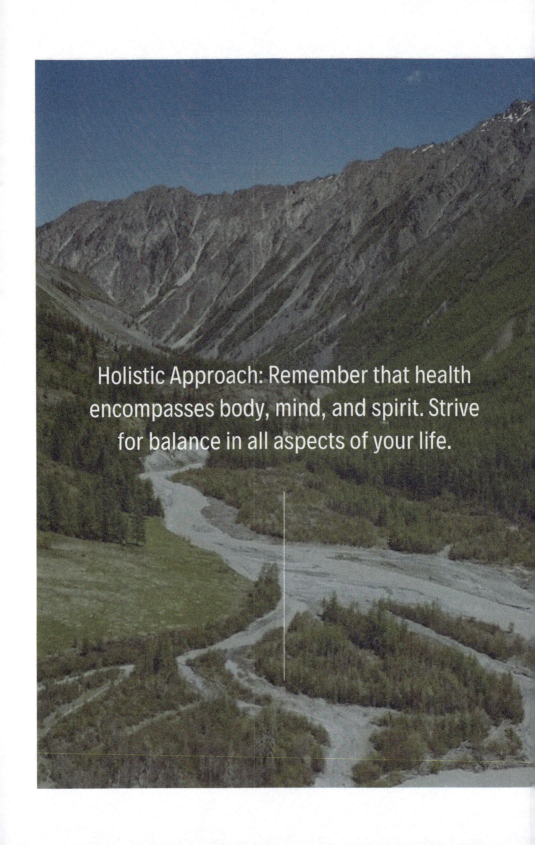

Holistic Approach: Remember that health encompasses body, mind, and spirit. Strive for balance in all aspects of your life.

"

"Nurture your spiritual connection.
A strong spiritual foundation can
provide strength and guidance in
your healing journey."- Barbara
O'Neill

@barbara.oneill.heals

LIKE, FOLLOW FOR MORE

Onion Feet Poultice Recipe – Inspired by Barbara O'Neill
Barbara O'Neill's holistic approach to health often incorporates natural remedies, and an onion poultice is one such remedy that she might recommend for its potential benefits. An onion poultice is believed to help draw out toxins, promote circulation, and offer relief for certain ailments, especially when applied to the feet. Here's a simple onion feet poultice recipe inspired by Barbara O'Neill's teachings:
Ingredients:
- 1 large onion (preferably organic)
- Thin cloth or muslin
- Bandage or adhesive tape

Instructions:
1. Prepare the Onion:
   - Peel the onion and cut it into thin slices. You can use either red or white onions for this poultice.
2. Steam the Onion Slices:
   - Place the onion slices in a steamer or a pot with a small amount of water. Steam the onion slices until they are softened but not overly cooked. This helps release the beneficial compounds within the onion.
3. Wrap the Onion Slices:
   - Lay the steamed onion slices on a clean, thin cloth or muslin. Arrange them in a single layer, leaving some space between each slice.
4. Fold and Secure:
   - Fold the cloth over the onion slices, creating a pouch or packet. Make sure the onion slices are securely wrapped within the cloth.
5. Test Temperature:
   - Before applying the poultice, test the temperature of the onion packet on the inside of your wrist to ensure it's comfortable and not too hot.
6. Apply to Feet:
   - Place the onion poultice on the soles of your feet. You can apply it to both feet or focus on a specific foot if needed.
7. Secure in Place:
   - Use a bandage or adhesive tape to secure the poultice in place on your feet. Make sure it's snug but not too tight.
8. Relax and Rest:
   - Keep the poultice on your feet for about 20–30 minutes. Relax and allow the natural properties of the onion to work.
9. Remove and Discard:
   - Gently remove the poultice from your feet and discard the used onion slices.
10. Cleanse Feet:
    - After removing the poultice, wash your feet with warm water to remove any onion residue and refresh your skin.

Remember that while onion poultices have been used for their potential benefits, individual responses may vary. If you have allergies or sensitive skin, it's advisable to test a small area before applying the poultice to your feet. As with any natural remedy, it's recommended to consult with a healthcare professional, especially if you have any existing health conditions or concerns.

Barbara O'Neill's Natural Headache Remedy

Barbara O'Neill's holistic approach to health often includes natural remedies that align with the body's innate healing mechanisms. For headaches, she might suggest a simple and soothing remedy that involves the use of essential oils and relaxation techniques. Here's a natural headache remedy inspired by Barbara O'Neill's teachings:

Ingredients:
- Peppermint essential oil
- Lavender essential oil
- Carrier oil (such as coconut oil or almond oil)
- Warm water
- Clean cloth or towel

Instructions:
1. Create a Relaxing Environment:
   - Find a quiet and comfortable space where you can relax and unwind.
2. Prepare a Bowl of Warm Water:
   - Fill a bowl with warm water. The temperature should be soothing and comfortable to the touch.
3. Essential Oil Blend:
   - In a small bowl, mix a few drops of peppermint essential oil and lavender essential oil with a carrier oil. The carrier oil helps dilute the essential oils and prevents skin irritation.
4. Head Massage:
   - Sit down and close your eyes. Gently massage a small amount of the essential oil blend onto your temples, forehead, and the base of your skull. Use gentle circular motions and apply light pressure.
5. Inhale and Relax:
   - Cup your hands over your nose and mouth, without touching your skin, and take slow, deep breaths. Inhale the soothing aroma of the essential oils. Allow the relaxing scent to help ease tension.
6. Warm Compress:
   - Dip a clean cloth or towel into the bowl of warm water. Wring out excess water and place the warm, damp cloth over your forehead or the back of your neck.
7. Rest and Breathe:
   - Close your eyes and take deep, slow breaths. Focus on the sensation of relaxation and let go of any tension.
8. Duration and Comfort:
   - Keep the warm compress on your forehead or neck for about 10-15 minutes, or until you feel relief.
9. Hydration and Rest:
   - Drink a glass of water to stay hydrated, as dehydration can contribute to headaches. Consider resting in a quiet space for a little while longer to support relaxation.

Barbara O'Neill's holistic headache remedy aims to provide a sense of relief through a combination of aromatherapy, massage, and relaxation techniques. Keep in mind that individual responses may vary, and this remedy is intended to complement, not replace, professional medical advice. If you experience severe or chronic headaches, it's recommended to consult a healthcare professional for proper diagnosis and treatment.

"Self Heal by Design" by Barbara O'Neill covers a wide range of general health tips and concepts that empower readers to take control of their well-being using natural and holistic approaches. Here are some of the general tips that the book might cover:

1. Holistic Approach:
   - Embrace a holistic approach that recognizes the interconnectedness of the mind, body, and spirit in achieving overall well-being.
2. Nutrient-Rich Diet:
   - Consume a diet rich in whole foods, emphasizing fruits, vegetables, whole grains, nuts, seeds, and lean proteins.
3. Hydration Importance:
   - Drink adequate water throughout the day to support proper bodily functions and assist in detoxification.
4. Mindful Eating:
   - Practice mindful eating by savoring each bite, eating slowly, and paying attention to hunger and fullness cues.
5. Stress Management:
   - Implement stress reduction techniques such as deep breathing, meditation, yoga, and spending time in nature.
6. Quality Sleep:
   - Prioritize consistent and restful sleep to support physical and mental rejuvenation.
7. Exercise Variety:
   - Engage in regular physical activity that includes a mix of cardiovascular exercise, strength training, and flexibility exercises.
8. Emotional Well-Being:
   - Cultivate emotional well-being by nurturing positive relationships, practicing gratitude, and engaging in activities that bring joy.
9. Natural Remedies:
   - Explore the potential benefits of herbs, essential oils, and other natural remedies to support health and healing.
10. Toxicity Reduction: – Minimize exposure to environmental toxins by choosing natural cleaning and personal care products.
11. Spiritual Connection: – Nurture your spiritual well-being through practices like meditation, prayer, and reflection.
12. pH Balance: – Understand the importance of maintaining a balanced pH level in the body through dietary choices and lifestyle.
13. Mind-Body Connection: – Recognize the influence of emotions on physical health and practice techniques to maintain emotional balance.
14. Preventive Care: – Take preventive measures to support the body's natural defenses and minimize the risk of illness.
15. Positive Mindset: – Cultivate a positive mindset that promotes self-care, self-love, and self-responsibility for health.
16. Natural Lifestyle: – Opt for natural and whole foods, avoiding processed and artificial ingredients as much as possible.
17. Self-Empowerment: – Empower yourself with knowledge about your body, health choices, and the impact of your lifestyle.

"Self Heal by Design" offers readers practical tools and insights to make informed decisions about their health and well-being. While these tips are a general overview, the book likely delves deeper into each topic, providing a comprehensive guide to living a balanced and healthy life.

99

Psalm 103:2-3 - "Praise the LORD, my soul, and forget not all his benefits—who forgives all your sins and heals all your diseases."

SAY – I COMMAND MY BODY
TO BE IN HEALTH.

99

"Seek community and support. Surround yourself with people who uplift and encourage you on your healing path." - Barbara O'Neill

@barbara.oneill.heals

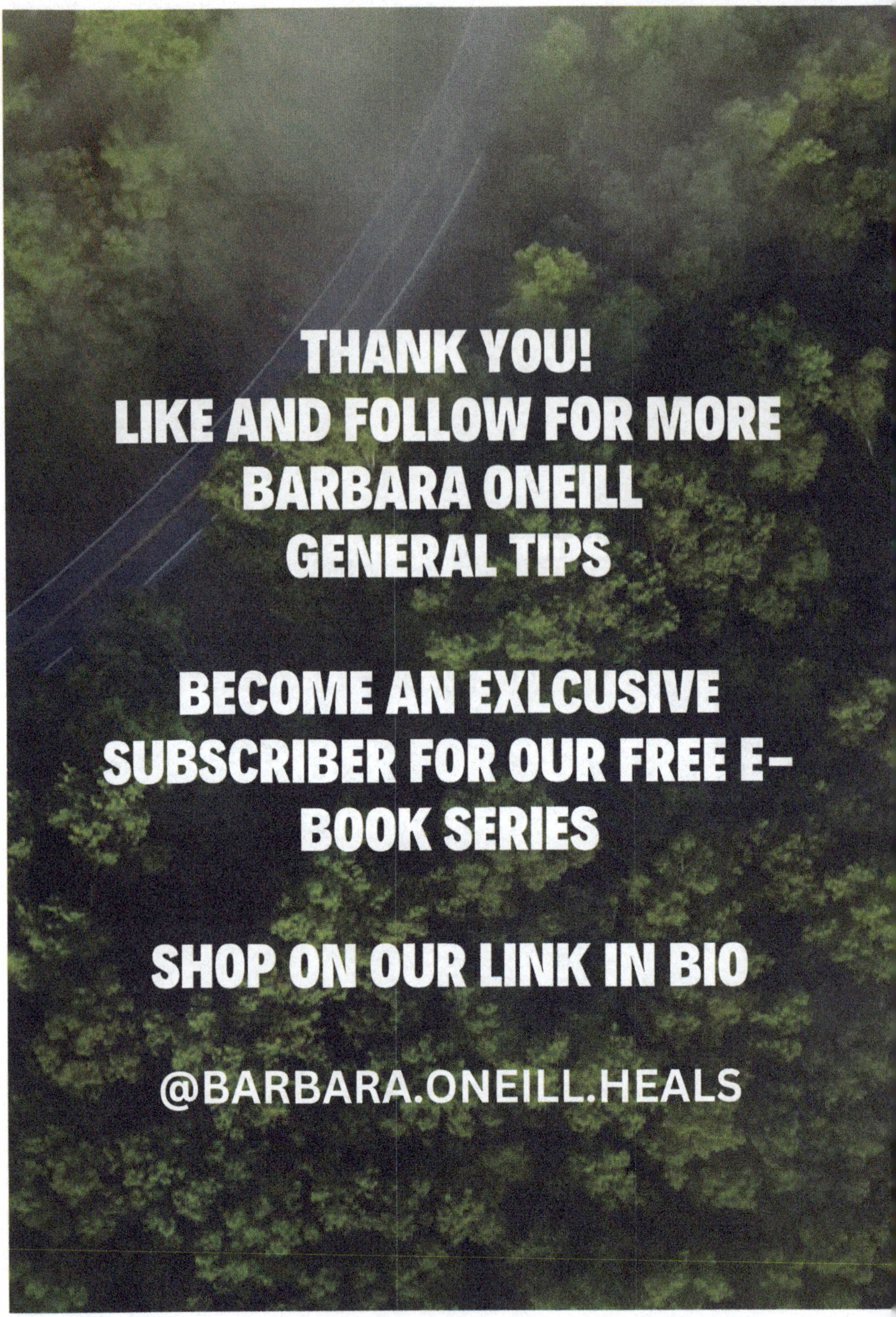
THANK YOU!
LIKE AND FOLLOW FOR MORE
BARBARA ONEILL
GENERAL TIPS
BECOME AN EXLCUSIVE
SUBSCRIBER FOR OUR FREE E-
BOOK SERIES
SHOP ON OUR LINK IN BIO
@BARBARA.ONEILL.HEALS

made with love:
"Do everything in love."

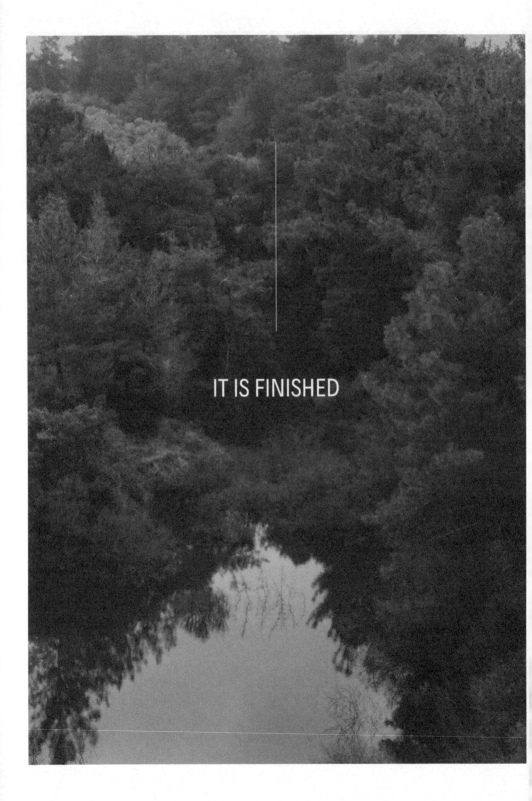

IT IS FINISHED

Made in the USA
Monee, IL
14 September 2023

42718115R00044